Yoga

Beginners Guide

For Yoga Poses
Easy Steps And
Pictures

Introduction

I want to thank you and congratulate you for downloading the book, *"Yoga: Beginners Guide - For Yoga Poses" - Easy Steps And Pictures*.

This book has easy to follow yoga poses and pictures you can use to practice yoga at home.

As Dr. Amit Ray, a spiritual master, aptly puts it, "Yoga is not a religion. It is a science, the science of well-being, youthfulness, integrating body, mind, and soul. The practice of Yoga aligns your body, mind and soul, keeps you mentally and physically fit, and helps you explore yourself in a better manner.

However, what exactly is yoga? How can you practice it, and how does it benefit you? These common questions pop into our mind whenever we hear someone rambling on about the amazingness of yoga.

This book seeks to answer these questions, as well as provide you with a step-by-step guide on how best to integrate various beneficial yoga poses into your everyday life and in the process, enhance your quality of life.

Let us begin our journey into yoga and your practice of it by gaining an in-depth insight of yoga as a mind and body practice.

Thanks again for downloading this book, I hope you enjoy it!

Table of Contents

Yoga: An In-Depth Understanding

As Yogi Bhagavad Gita said in one of his teachings, "Yoga is the journey of the self, through the self, to the self."

Generally, most of us are accustomed to seeking fulfillment from things and people in our immediate surroundings and hardly perceive fulfillment as an inner feeling. Nevertheless, different experiences we go through help us understand that no external factor has the potential to fulfill our deep longing for satisfaction and fulfilment. Unfortunately, most of us often gravitate towards action instead of awareness. In this state, we lack awareness of our surroundings, the present, and ourselves which is why we are never fully content with our lives or ourselves.

As a practice, Yoga helps you achieve a state of total calmness, tranquility, and contentment. Yoga is the ultimate answer to the longing, yearning, and chaos we feel inside, and outside us. So, what exactly is yoga?

Yoga is a practice that reverses the routine outward energy flow and consciousness, making your mind the dynamic hub of perception; allowing it to stop reliance on your fallible senses, and become capable of properly experiencing the truth.

Yoga is a mental, spiritual, and physical discipline that originated sometime in the fifth and sixth centuries BCE in India. The term 'yoga' comes from the word 'yuj', a Sanskrit word meaning 'to bind' or 'to yoke'. A common interpretation of yoga is as discipline or union. Male and female yoga practitioners bear the names 'yogi' and 'yogini', respectively.

Yoga unites your body, mind, and soul by making use of the eight yoga sutras; sutras are the eight elements in your body that can help you attain enlightenment.

Yoga Sutras

Yoga sutras, also referred to as the eight-limbed path or eight-fold path are as follows:

1. The Yamas

The first sutra is the 'Yamas' which are the behavior patterns or ethical standards describing how you need to live your life. The Yamas include 'ahimsa' which means practicing non-violence and not harming anyone, 'Satya' which means being truthful, 'Asteya' which translates to not stealing anything from anyone, 'bramacharya' which refers to exercising self-restraint, and 'aparigraha' which refers to non-covetousness.

2. The Niyamas

Niyamas are the second Sutra, and refer to developing an attitude of self-discipline. The Niyamas set guidelines for healthy, clean, and good living. They include 'Saucha' which means cleanliness, 'Samtosha' which refers to contentment and being modest, 'tapas' meaning cleansing your body of impurities and staying healthy, 'svadhyaya' which translates to 'self-inquiry' and lastly, 'isvara pranidhana' meaning surrendering to your God.

3. Asanas

The third factor is 'Asanas' which are the physical positions practiced in yoga. Your body serves as a temple for your spirit, which is why it is your duty to care of it, and ensure it always remains healthy and in a fit state. By practicing various Asanas, you can purify and detoxify your body, and enhance your ability to properly focus, meditate, and concentrate.

4. Pranayama

Pranayama is the fourth sutra, which means controlling your breathing. By regulating your breathing movements with the help of breathing exercises, you make the best use of 'prana', the energy living inside you. By doing so, it rejuvenates your body, and increases your average lifespan.

5. Pratyahara

Pratyahara is the fifth sutra; it means directing your attention inward. Practicing Pratyahara helps you realistically understand yourself through observing your habits, cravings, and desires, and is thus able to eliminate all negative traits from your personality.

6. Dharana

Dharana, the sixth sutra, refers to concentrating on your mind with proper focus and energy. By concentrating on one thing in particular, it helps augment your focus and the ability to be attentive on just one thing at a time.

7. Dhyana

The seventh sutra, dhyana, refers to contemplation or meditation. Meditation helps you attain stillness and calmness, which gives you further and better insight into your mind.

8. Samadhi

Samadhi is the eighth sutra and refers to a state characterized by continual ecstasy or bliss. This state commonly refers to as state of enlightenment, where you make good use of all the seven sutras mentioned above, and are able to derive the benefits they offer to acquire nirvana. If you devote to the regular practice of yoga, strive to achieve perfection in it and explore it deeper, you will be able to objectify the state of nirvana.

Yoga As A Way Of Life

Contrary to popular belief, yoga is deficient of strong religious ties. Yoga is a way of life that helps you improve your quality of life, and acquire peacefulness in every aspect of life. People belonging to different religions across the globe practice yoga to deepen their spiritual and religious beliefs, and achieve a state of complete awareness and serenity.

Physical yoga commonly practiced worldwide is hatha yoga. Hatha yoga is a combination of sun and moon postures. Sun postures are heating postures (postures that heat up your body), while moon postures are postures that cool down your body. By using hatha yoga, you energize, as well as calm down your body.

This guide is going to shed some light on different hatha yoga postures and practices. By engaging in, and practicing these poses, you will enjoy the following benefits:

Stress, Anxiety, and Depression Relief: Yoga helps you connect to the portions of your brain responsible for regulating stress; by tapping into these areas of your brain and exercising them, you gain complete freedom from stress, anxiety, and depression.

- **Lose Weight:** Yoga energizes your body and enhances your metabolism. When your metabolic rate enhances, you burn calories at a faster pace, a fastened heart rate is a critical factor in healthy weight.

- **Become Happier:** By eliminating stress from your life and body, you become calmer which improves your emotional well-being, making you feel happier. Moreover, different yoga poses improve serotonin levels in your body (serotonin is a mood-boosting hormone). This enhances your state of happiness.

- **Improve Your Health**: Various yoga poses reduce inflammation in the body, stabilize your blood cholesterol and sugar levels, detoxify your body, regulate your blood pressure, and keep your heart healthy. All these factors improve your immune system and health, keeping various serious bodily ailments and disorders at bay.

- **Focus Better:** By practicing yoga postures aimed at enhancing your concentration, you can improve your focus and attention span. This helps you efficiently manage your time and increase productivity.

- **Become More Creative:** By using various yoga poses designed to improve your thinking and creative abilities, you can improve your innovative skills and become better at coming up with unique ideas.

- **Builds Strength, Muscles, and Protects Your Bones:** By performing different yoga poses aimed at enhancing your physical and muscular strength, you build more muscle mass, and strengthen your bone; this reduces bone loss, tissue inflammation, and keeps you safe from conditions such as arthritis.

- **Yoga Improves Your Body Posture:** Most physical problems stem from having a bad posture. Yoga can easily correct this problem. All yoga poses help improve your body posture and when you correct your posture, your physical health improves.

- **Yoga Combats Insomnia and Sleep Related Problems:** In addition to the aforementioned benefits, by reducing stress, improving your well-being, and enhancing your calmness, yoga cures insomnia and treats various sleep related problems.

- **Yoga Increases Self-Esteem and Confidence:** Yoga helps you understand yourself better, gives you peace of mind, and gets rid of negative, poisonous thoughts that lower your self-worth and confidence. When these changes take place in your body, your self-esteem, and confidence start perking up.

- **Yoga Improves Your Awareness:** Yoga gives you a chance to be cognizant of the present and value it. Moreover, it improves your awareness and mindfulness, which helps you live a better life.

To enjoy these benefits, start practicing yoga today! In the next few sections, we shall outline different yoga poses you can practice to improve your quality of life.

Stress, Anxiety, And Depression Relief: Easy Yoga Poses

Yoga is an amazing stress reliever. It eases all anxiety and depression symptoms. It transfers your attention to your breath and body, which reduces anxiety. The yoga poses discussed below curb anxiety, depression, and stress. You can perform them in the order described below, or execute them individually, as you please.

Anjali Mudra

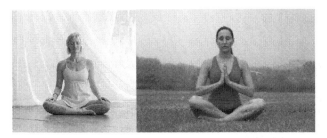

Anjali mudra, also known as salutation seal is a great way to induce a relaxed, meditative state of consciousness and awareness that diverts your focus from all thoughts that trigger stress and anxiety.

Mudra refers to hand positions. In yoga, different nerves in your hands connect to various parts of your brain. By building a connection with those portions, you can produce various desired results.

Anjali mudra is practiced with your hands in front of your heart or heart chakra (a chakra is a point of spiritual power in your body) this helps you establish harmony between the left and right side of your body, thus stabilizing your emotions, which curtails anxiety and stress.

How to Perform It

To practice it, follow the steps below:

1. Sit in a comfortable pose and cross your legs (if this is comfortable). You could open or close your eyes as convenient. However, for starters, it is best to close your eyes to limit external distractions.

2. Bring your hands to the center of your chest and join them together.

3. Maintain this pose for about ten minutes, and try to relax. Increase your duration by one minute after every two days until you can practice it for 20 to 30 minutes. Performing it regularly will easily reduce stress.

MarjaryAsana

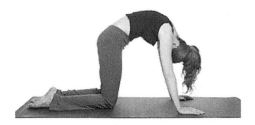

Maryjaryasana, also the cat pose, is a great way to massage your entire body and relax it. It massages your belly organs and spine, and busts away all stress. It also improves your overall health as it stimulates your digestive tract, as well as the spinal fluid.

How to Perform It

1. To perform the cat pose, get on the floor and kneel.

2. Extend your legs backwards and keep your arms straight.

3. Curve your back a little and lower down your head to relax. If you are a beginner, take care when maintaining this pose and place your wrists under your shoulders and your knees right below the hips, so that your alignment is perfect.

4. Maintain this pose for five to fifteen minutes, or for as long as is convenient for you. If you are a beginner, doing it for six minutes in three intervals of two minutes each is sufficient and very effective. As you progress, you can increase its duration.

Uttana Shishosana

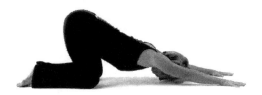

Also known as the extended puppy pose, uttana shishosana is an effective stress relieving pose. It lengthens your spine, calms down your active mind and relaxes your entire body. It eliminates the signs of chronic tension, insomnia, and stress.

How to Perform It

1. To perform the extended puppy pose, kneel on the ground.

2. Open your hips, extend your arms forward, and place them on the floor. Hold this pose for about five to ten minutes.

3. Novices can execute the pose for one minute, take a break, and then do it for a minute more. Start increasing its duration with the passage of time.

Practice these poses every day, or set one pose for one day and do another on the second day and so on. Within two weeks, you will start experiencing amazing results on your stress, anxiousness, and depression.

Weight Loss Yoga Asanas

Yoga is an amazing calorie burner and fat buster. It is particularly effective at fighting stubborn fat reserves that sneakily build up in your body after you reach the age of 40. Various studies conducted on the benefits of yoga have shown that yoga lowers the levels of various stress hormones, promotes insulin sensitivity, and augments your metabolic rate–all these changes work as signals to make your body burn fat at a faster rate.

Here are some wonderful and effective yoga poses that can help you lose weight easily, quickly, successfully, and in a healthy manner.

Anjaneyasana

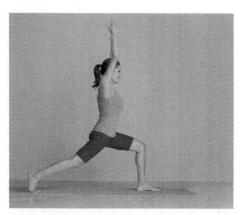

Also known as the crescent pose, Anjaneyasana is effective at firming your thighs, abs and hips, and losing the tough fat lodged in these parts. It fortifies your gluteus muscles, quadriceps, and your abdomen. It is excellent for relieving sciatica pain. Moreover, it expands your shoulders, lungs, and chest and enhances your stamina, concentration, core awareness, and balance. It is simple and easy to practice, which makes it perfect for beginners.

How to Perform It

1. To engage in this pose, stand straight with your feet together, arms at your sides, and toes forward.

2. Now, inhale and slowly raise your arms over your head. Extend your fingertips towards the ceiling.

3. Exhale and then bend forward. Bring your hands to the floor. You can bend your knees if you are a beginner.

4. Inhale and when you start exhaling, step your right leg backwards into the lunge pose. Keep your left knee bent to about 90 degrees. Inhale and gently raise your arms overhead and gaze forward. Maintain this pose for five to ten seconds and then return to the starting pose. Repeat these cycle five to ten times.

Virabhadrasana

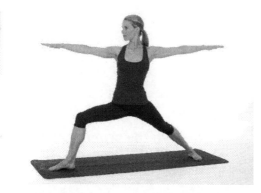

Warrior pose, or Virabhadrasana is an excellent yoga pose for stretching your back, strengthening your tummy, buttocks and thighs, and for losing annoying body fat. This pose is not suitable for people suffering from high blood pressure, back or knee pain, and any sort of condition pertinent to the limbs or joints.

How to Perform It

1. To execute the warrior pose, stand straight with both your feet together. Keep your hands by the sides.

2. Now, slowly extend the right leg a little forward and extend your left one backwards.

3. Bend the right knee gently, so you enter the lunge pose. Now, slowly twist your torso a little, so you face the bent right leg.

4. Turn the left foot sideways and exhale. Straighten both your arms and slowly raise your body upwards and slightly away from the bent knee. Stretch the arms upwards.

5. Gently tilt the torso a little backwards to arch your back. Maintain this pose for ten seconds.

6. To exit the pose, exhale and then straighten the right knee. Push the right leg to return to the starting position. Be very gentle when exiting so you do not injure your legs.

Repeat it with the other leg. You can do it for ten minutes in the start and increase its duration with time. Watch this helpful video to understand how to do this pose.

Surya Namaskar

Popularly known as sun salutation, surya namaskar is a series of different yoga Asanas carried out in succession. It has an amazing effect on weight loss as it makes use of lots of backward and forward bending Asanas that stretch and flex your spinal column, giving your entire body a profound stretch. This asana is a complete body workout that strengthens and works out every muscle in your body, promoting total body weight loss.

How to Perform It

Here's what you need to do to perform the sun salutation (images below)

1. Begin in the prayer pose or pranamasana. Stand straight with your feet together. Balance your body and weight on your feet. Open your chest and gently relax the shoulders. Inhale and lift your arms up. Now, exhale and gently bring forward your palms and unite them in front of your chest.

2. Next, get into the hasta Uttanasana or raised arms pose. Breathe in and lift your arms up and backwards. Keep your biceps close to your ears

3. Now perform hasta padasana or hand-to-foot pose. Breathe out and bend forward. Keep your spine erect. Slowly bring your hands to the ground besides your feet.

4. After that, execute the ashwasanchalasana or equestrian pose. To do it, breathe in and push the right leg backwards. Bring your right knee towards the ground and then look upwards.

5. Next, perform the Dandasana or stick pose. To perform it, breathe in, and take your left leg backwards, straightening your entire body.

6. Now, perform the Ashtanganamaskara known as salutation with eight parts. Gently bring the knees down towards the floor. Start exhaling. Take your hips backwards and slide forward. Rest the chest and your chin on the ground. Raise your buttocks a little and arch them. Your hands, knees, feet, chin, and chest should touch the ground.

7. Next, perform the Bhujaangasana or cobra pose. Slide forward. Now, raise your chest upwards to form the cobra pose. You can keep your elbows bent and shoulders slightly away from your ears.

8. After that, perform the Parvatasana, also known as the mountain pose. To do it, breathe out and lift your hips and your tailbone upwards. Maintain a V shaped posture.

9. Next, perform the equestrian pose, hasta padasana pose, and Hasta Uttanasana pose. We have described these poses above, so follow those guidelines to perform them.

10. End the sun salutation with the Tadasana pose. Exhale and straighten your body. Bring your arms down. Relax and analyze the various sensations taking place in your body.

Carry out these amazing poses and soon, you will experience a remarkable weight reduction.

Follow the image sequence below

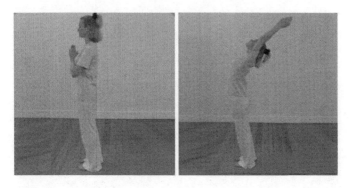

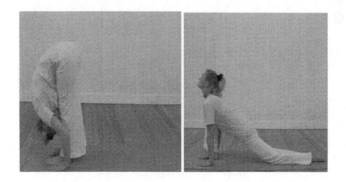

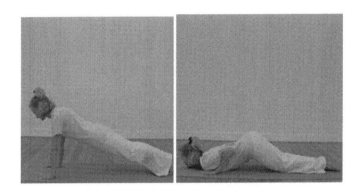

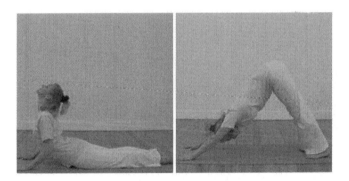

Happiness Yoga Asanas

Life throws many curveballs our way; this often makes it difficult to stay happy all the time; still, a life devoid of happiness, is meaningless. By practicing yoga, you can easily improve your state of well-being and happiness, and restore tranquility and joy back into your life. Below are a few great poses that can help you become happy and amplify your happiness.

Goddess Pose

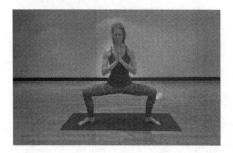

The goddess pose, or utkatakonasana, is one of the most effective happiness inducing yoga poses. The goddess pose is an empowering and energizing pose that stretches your chest, groin, and hips, helps you lose weight, improves blood circulation, and augments the serotonin levels in your body, consequently improving your mood.

How to Perform It

1. To perform this pose, first enter the mountain pose.

2. Now, stand up and keep your arms at the sides.

3. Place your hands on the hips. Turn towards the right and step both feet about four feet apart. Slightly turn the toes outwards, exhale and bend the knees over the toes.

4. Lower the hips and enter the squat position. Try bringing your hips as parallel as possible to the floor.

5. Extend the arms towards the sides and keep the palms faced downwards. Spiral the thumbs upwards towards the roof and move the palms forward.

6. Bend the elbows and then point the fingertips towards the roof. Keep your forearms and upper arms at a 90-degree angle.

7. Tuck the tailbone in lightly. Press the buttocks forward and keep the knees and toes aligned. Hold for ten breaths.

8. Slowly, return the hands to your buttocks and keep the spine upright. Straighten the legs and step back your feet together. Relax and take a few deep breaths.

Practice this pose for five to ten minutes daily to escalate your happiness level

Adho Mukha Savanasana

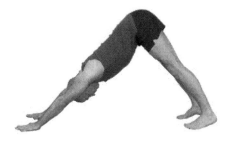

Downward Facing Dog, also known as adho mukha savanasana, is an excellent pose for curbing unnecessary and incessant mood swings and changing gloominess into happiness. In addition, it improves bone density, enhances blood circulation, eliminates back pain, stiffness, and increases your flexibility.

How to Perform It

1. Begin on all fours. Your hands should be beneath your shoulders and the palms should press onto the floor.

2. Tuck the toes under. Now, slowly lift the knees off the ground as you gently straighten the legs.

3. Maintain the pose for five to ten breaths. Practice it daily to elevate your mood and stay happy.

In addition to the above poses, the surya namaskar also improves your mental well-being and reduces mood swings.

Fitness and Optimum Health Asanas

Unless you are in good health, it is impossible to enjoy all of life's little pleasures. Staying healthy is one of our top priorities. Yoga can easily help you accomplish this goal. Below are brilliant yoga poses guaranteed to improve your health and help you manage problems such as inflammation, heart conditions, blood pressure, diabetes, and other issues of that sort.

Om Mantra

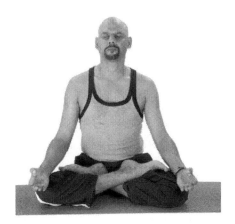

Om mantra is a fantastic yoga pose that helps cure migraines, tension, high blood pressure, constipation, indigestion, gastric problems, and inflammation, and reduce the likelihood of suffering from a heart attack. Moreover, you can use it to overcome stammering, and build your confidence. It also improves your mental awareness and internal brightness.

How to Perform It

1. Start by sitting in an easy pose or Sukhasana. For that, you need to place your right leg over the left one or vice versa.

2. Now, close your eyes.

3. Place the hands forward in Gyan mudra. To perform the Gyan mudra, keep your hand

open and place it on your knees. Now, touch the tips of the thumb and index finger and straighten the remaining three fingers.

4. Keep your neck and back straight. Make sure to keep all your body muscles in a relaxed state, and sit as still as possible.

5. Take a deep breath and say 'Om' loudly. Concentrate on the word 'Om' only, relax your mind, and rid it of all its worries. Do it for five minutes in the beginning, and slowly increase its duration to 25 minutes in about a month or so. Doing it daily enables you to become incredibly fit and strong.

Dhanurasana

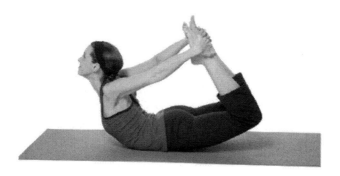

Bow pose, or Dhanurasana is great at improving digestion and curbing digestion related problems, including acidity and gastric reflux. It massages your liver and abdominal muscles, and organs that stimulate your gastric secretions, thus improving the digestion process. It also helps in controlling and curing diabetes, neck and back pains, hormonal imbalances and menstrual disorders.

Note: Individuals suffering from hernia, slipped disc, and colitis should avoid practicing this pose.

How to Perform It

1. Lie completely flat on your stomach. Keep the feet and legs together. Your arms should be besides your body.

2. Bend your knees. Bring your heels near your buttocks.

3. Place your chin gently on the ground. Clasp your hand around your ankles.

4. Inhale deeply and raise the head trunk along with the legs above the floor, so you can lift your legs. Raise your legs slightly or higher if convenient for you.

5. Pull the legs and hands in opposite directions. Support your body on the ground.

6. Maintain this pose for at least five breaths, or for as long as is convenient for you.

7. To exit the pose, slowly relax your limbs and head to the beginning position. Doing it thrice daily can help you attain all the aforementioned benefits.

Chandra Bhedana

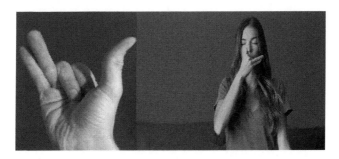

Moon breath or Chandra bhedana is an excellent pose for combatting insomnia and initiating sleep easily. Moreover, it helps cool down your body, which makes it effective at fighting stress and anger problems.

Your left nostril links with your body's ability to cool down, while the right one associates with heating. Chandra bhedana focuses on using the left nostril to produce a cooling effect on your body and mind. This energy massages your organs activating your sleep. In addition, it signals the vagus nerve to trigger the 'calmness-inducing' portions of your brain, which helps you become relaxed and peaceful.

How to Perform It

1. To perform this asana, sit comfortably on the floor, yoga mat, or a chair.

2. Make Mrigi mudra or deer seal using your right hand. To make it, bend the middle and index fingers in your palm and extend the pinky and ring fingers.

3. Now, press the right thumb on the right nostril and inhale via the left nostril.

4. Release the right thumb. Take the ring finger to your left nostril and breathe out via the right nostril. Continue this practice for one to three minutes, or until you begin feeling calm. Practicing it daily allows you to sleep comfortably.

In addition to these poses, all the poses discussed in the other chapters help improve your health too. Downward facing dog and sun salutation are great for managing arthritis and increasing bone density.

Yoga Poses For Increasing Confidence, Inner Peace, Awareness, And Creativity

Confidence, inner peace, awareness, and creativity are key factors required to gain the strength, courage, and the ability to pursue your goals and actualize them. Moreover, these traits enhance your sense of well-being and help you feel good about yourself. The good thing is that yoga can help you attain all these traits.

Below are brilliant yoga poses you can use to enhance self-esteem, self-confidence, innovative skills, and awareness.

Chair Pose for Boosting Confidence

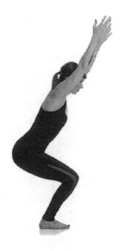

Chair pose, or Utkatasana energize your body and boost your self-esteem, self-worth, and confidence. Moreover, it is amazingly effective at stretching your legs and thighs, and strengthening the muscles in these parts. In addition, it promotes weight loss.

How to Perform It

1. Start in the mountain pose and keep your feet at hip width apart.

2. Inhale and extend your arms parallel to the ground. Your palms should face downwards.

3. Exhale and then bend your knees to form the squat position.

4. Lower your hips and move them backwards as if you are sitting in a chair. Your hips should be higher than your knees.

5. Press your shoulder down. Try arching your spine and then relax your shoulders.

6. Maintain this pose for five to ten breaths.

7. To exit the pose, inhale and then gently press down into your feet to straighten your legs. Inhale and raise the arms upward and exhale to release them downwards. Practice this pose daily to augment your self-confidence by manifolds.

Child's Pose to Become Innovative and Peaceful

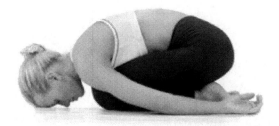

Children have amazing imagination, which is why the child's pose or Shishuasana helps you become extremely imaginative and creative. Moreover, it improves your consciousness and helps you relax, which allows you to acquire inner peace.

Additionally, it strengthens your back and relieves you of all sorts of backaches. Moreover, it is an excellent pose for improving your digestion and eliminating problems associated with poor digestion. Practice it regularly.

How to Perform It

1. Begin on all fours. Start relaxing and then spread the knees wide apart.

2. Rest the buttocks on the heels.

3. Sit up, lengthen the spine via the crown part of your head, and inhale.

4. Exhale and bow forward. Drape the torso between the thighs. Make sure that the chest and heart rests between the thighs, or on top of them.

5. Let the forehead rest on the floor.

6. Extend your arms forward with the palms facing downwards.

7. Press your back slightly, so your buttocks connect with the heels. Lengthen as much as you possibly can.

8. Let all sort of tension drain away from your body.

9. Keep your eyes closed and focus on your breath only.

10. Maintain this pose for 30 to 40 seconds in the start and take it up to 20 to 30 minutes with time.

11. To get up from the pose, walk your torso upwards with your hands and sit on the heels.

Hakini Mudra for Increased Awareness, Inner Peace, Improved Concentration, and Better Memory

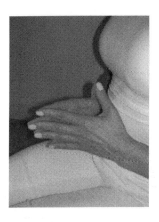

Hakini mudra is extremely effective at enhancing your concentration, awareness, mindfulness of thoughts, attaining inner peace, and boosting your memory. It activates your sixth chakra, which lies on your forehead, which is associated with intuition and mental awareness. In addition, it balances your brain's left and right hemispheres, which improves your power to retain and memorize information.

How to Perform It

1. To perform it, sit in the easy pose as discussed earlier.

2. Now, bring your hands forward and touch the right and left thumbs together.

3. Gently, touch the fingertips of all the fingers on both your hands.

4. Spread the fingers apart.

5. Practice it for at least ten minutes daily and you can increase its duration to up to 60 minutes, or even more. The more you practice it, the better your concentration becomes. Moreover, it helps you become increasingly mindful of the present and enjoy it.

To become peaceful, calm, and confident, regularly exercise all these poses. You can alternate different poses on different days, so you can enjoy the benefits of all the poses discussed in this book.

Important Tips

Remember one thing clearly: consistency is the key to success. Therefore, be consistent in your practice of yoga and practice it daily. Of course, you cannot do each pose mentioned in this book daily, so stick with a few for one to two weeks, and then try new ones; or you could perform poses depending on your need. For instance, if you are facing chronic digestion and back pain problems, you could engage in poses relevant to these issues for a month, or until your problem vanishes.

Some poses, or all poses may appear difficult in the beginning especially if you live a sedentary lifestyle. That does not mean you should give up. It means you must keep going until you perfect every pose. Remember, great things come to those who wait and with time, so the more time you devote to your yoga practice, the better you will become at it. Try your hand at yoga and unlock an amazing life.

Conclusion

Yoga, if practiced regularly can help you live a harmonious and beautiful life. Use the yoga poses described in this book to become healthy, happy, and calm.

Thank you again for downloading this book!

I hope this book was able to help you to know all that you need to know about yoga as a beginner.

The next step is to start practicing what you have learnt and see a change in your life.

Finally, would you be kind enough to leave a review for this book on Amazon.

Click here to leave a review for this book on Amazon!

Or go here:

http://www.amazon.com/dp/B01BMK5D7G

Thank you and good luck!

PS: Look at the next page with more information on upcoming books!

Preview Of - Smoothies Cleanse - Detox Diet And Lose Weight In A Healthy Way

This book will provide you with comprehensive information about smoothie cleanse.

Losing weight is a challenge for many people. That is why with each passing day, there is a new diet claiming that it can help you lose weight. Unfortunately, many of these diet plans fall short of the hype they are often associated with. They tend to work for the first few days then after some time, you get to a weight loss plateau where you just cannot seem to move forward towards your weight loss plans. Then you may ask yourself. Why do they fall short of whatever it is they promise when they seem to be very good on paper? Well, while there may be many reasons as to why you may struggle losing weight, it is important to understand that if you want to start losing weight fast, you need to start by detoxifying your body of all toxins.

Detoxification helps to eliminate toxic overload from your body and makes it easier to lose weight. This is because toxins are stored in the fat cells, and the more toxins you have, the more the fat cells expand making it harder to lose weight even as you reduce your calorie intake.

For effective weight loss, it is important to first eliminate these toxins through detoxification before going on any weight loss program. Smoothies are not only good for eliminating excess toxins in the body; they also help to heal the body and improve overall health and wellness.

In this book, you will find a detailed guide to help you achieve quick and effective weight loss through detoxification and fat loss. It would also teach you how to eat healthy and train your body to naturally start craving healthy foods.

[Click here to check out the rest of "Smoothies Cleanse - Detox Diet And Lose Weight In A Healthy Way".](#)

Or go to: http://amzn.to/1L7Yxmg

Made in the USA
Columbia, SC
08 December 2017